FAMILIES IN
THE ICU

FAMILIES IN THE ICU

A Survival Guide

DR. MELANIE TIDMAN

Library of Congress Control Number:		2015913430
ISBN:	Hardcover	978-1-5035-9930-7
	Softcover	978-1-5035-9929-1
	eBook	978-1-5035-9928-4

Print information available on the last page.

Rev. date: 08/18/2015

To order additional copies of this book, contact:
Xlibris
1-888-795-4274
www.Xlibris.com
Orders@Xlibris.com
714296

CONTENTS

From the Author vii

Definitions 1

Review of Brain Function 9

The Injury... 17

Roles of Medical Personnel in the Icu 23

Terminology 29

Flow Sheet of Possible Discharge Options and Nurse-to-
Patient Ratios... 45

Frequently Asked Questions for Your Doctor or Medical Staff....47

Community and Online Resources..............................51

References...57

FROM THE AUTHOR

This book has grown out of my own experience as a family member of a critically ill patient in the intensive care unit (ICU) and my thirty-six years' experience working with ICU families. Even with my background as a health-care provider, faced with this situation, I found myself confused, frustrated, exhausted, and afraid. I needed a handy resource that would provide crucial information, definitions, and explanations to allow me to communicate more effectively with medical personnel about the care of my loved one.

This book was written for families of patients who have been admitted to an intensive care unit and who may have been diagnosed with either a stroke or a traumatic brain injury (TBI). However, the information contained within these pages may prove useful to family members of patients in the ICU with a variety of diagnoses.

The intention of this book is to provide information to assist families with the care of their family member and to foster good communication with medical personnel. The book is based on a book, developed in part by actual ICU families and myself, as part of a doctoral research study to measure the level of satisfaction with care and communication between family members and the medical personnel who serve them. Results of the study suggested that family satisfaction with care and communication improved because of the information contained in the book.

It is hoped that this book will contain valuable information for family members and will provide a resource to answer questions regarding the care of ICU patients with TBI or stroke. It is also hoped that this book will assist families in communicating more effectively with medical staff in order to ultimately benefit the care of the patient and improve patient outcomes.

Melanie McCormick Tidman DHSc, MA, OTR/L

DEFINITIONS

def·i·ni·tion n. 1.
The teacher gave de
of the new words.

GENERAL DEFINITIONS

TRAUMATIC BRAIN INJURY

Traumatic brain injury (TBI) can occur as a result of external physical force to the head, which can produce altered states of consciousness (altered mental status or AMS) and physical, psychological, behavioral, or emotional impairments. These impairments may be temporary or permanent. TBI can occur in infants, children, adolescents, and adults. Some causes of TBI are motor vehicle accidents, assaults, falls, sports injuries, explosions, shaken baby trauma, and bicycle and pedestrian accidents. TBI can be mild or severe. Examples of mild TBI may be a concussion where there is no loss of consciousness or visible physical injury. Even if a TBI is mild, it may still cause temporary or permanent changes in the way someone feels, acts, and interacts with those around them.

ACQUIRED BRAIN INJURY

Acquired brain injury (ABI) is caused by an internal condition such as a stroke, lack of oxygen (anoxia), brain tumor, or exposure to toxic substances. Signs and symptoms are very similar to those of TBI with either temporary or permanent effects on a person's level of function. (Some associated terms can be seen in the "terminology" section of this book, which may include subarachnoid hemorrhage, subdural/epidural hematoma, etc.) A more formal definition of brain injury found on the state of New Mexico Mi Via program website is as follows:

Brain injury means an injury to the brain of traumatic or acquired origin, resulting in total or

3

partial functional disability, psychosocial impairment, or both. The term applies to open and closed head injuries caused by an insult to the brain from an outside physical force; anoxia, electrical shock, shaken baby syndrome; toxic and chemical substances; near drowning; infections; tumors, or vascular accidents. TBI/ABI may be temporary or permanent, partial or total impairments in one or more areas including, but not limited to cognition; language; memory; attention; reasoning; abstract thinking; judgment; problem solving; sensory, perceptual, and motor abilities; psychosocial behavior; physical function; information processing; and speech. (www.mivianm. org)

STATISTICS

According to the Centers for Disease Control and Prevention (CDC), in the year 2001 alone, five hundred thousand Americans suffered from TBI; and every year, at least 1.7 million TBIs occur either by itself or in combination with other injuries (www.cdc. gov/TraumaticBrainInjury/statistics.html). Total combined rates of TBI-related hospitalizations, ED visits, and deaths climbed slowly from a rate of 521.0 per one hundred thousand in 2001 to 615.7 per one hundred thousand in 2005. The rates then dipped to 595.1 per one hundred thousand in 2006 and 566.7 per one hundred thousand in 2007. The rates then spiked sharply in 2008 and continued to climb through 2010 to a rate of 823.7 per one hundred thousand. Of the cases studied, alcohol is a significant influencing factor in about 50 percent of all TBI cases; males between the ages of fifteen and twenty-four are more likely to sustain a TBI, abuse/ assault count for 64 percent of all TBI cases with falls being the major cause of TBI among children and the elderly (www.cdc.gov/ TraumaticBrainInjury/statistics.html).

STROKE

Brain Stroke

Ischemic Stroke   *Hemorrhagic Stroke*

Blockage of blood vessels; lack of blood flow to affected area   Rupture of blood vessels; leakage of blood

Stroke is the third leading cause of death in the United States. Each year, there are a total of eight hundred thousand strokes, of which approximately two hundred thousand are recurrent strokes. Thus, secondary prevention of ischemic stroke remains a good treatment strategy. Secondary prevention is specifically targeted toward modifiable risk factors (Ferri, 2015).

Risk Factors for Stroke

Age is the most important risk factor. Modifiable risk factors include hypertension (high blood pressure), hyperlipidemia (high fat content in the blood), cigarette smoking, excessive alcohol consumption, physical inactivity, obesity (i.e., a body mass index of >25 kg/m^2), and diabetes mellitus.

Physical Findings and Clinical Presentation

Stroke presents itself in many ways. Typically, the individual has a sudden definable loss of motor, sensory, visual, or cognitive functions that have a clear time of onset and that are noticed by others or by the individuals themselves. Physical findings—such as weakness and/or numbness in one limb or on one side of the body, facial droop, visual field loss, or the inability to understand or communicate with others—raise one's suspicion of a stroke event (Ferri, 2015).

Etiology (Causes of Stroke)

Strokes are generally divided into ischemic or hemorrhagic (i.e., intraparenchymal or subarachnoid hemorrhage).

Ischemic strokes are caused by large-vessel atherosclerosis (buildup of plaques on the inside of the arteries); cardioembolism, which is a clot forming as a result of a rhythm condition such as in atrial fibrillation (a rhythm disorder of the heart) or cardiomyopathy; or small-vessel disease, such as lacunar stroke. Rare causes such as recreational drug use (e.g., cocaine abuse), arterial dissection, and hypercoagulable states (too much clotting factor in the blood) need to be considered when ischemic stroke occurs in younger individuals.

The most common cause of intracerebral hemorrhage is uncontrolled hypertension. Spontaneous rupture of a brain aneurysm causes subarachnoid hemorrhage.

NOTES

REVIEW OF BRAIN FUNCTION

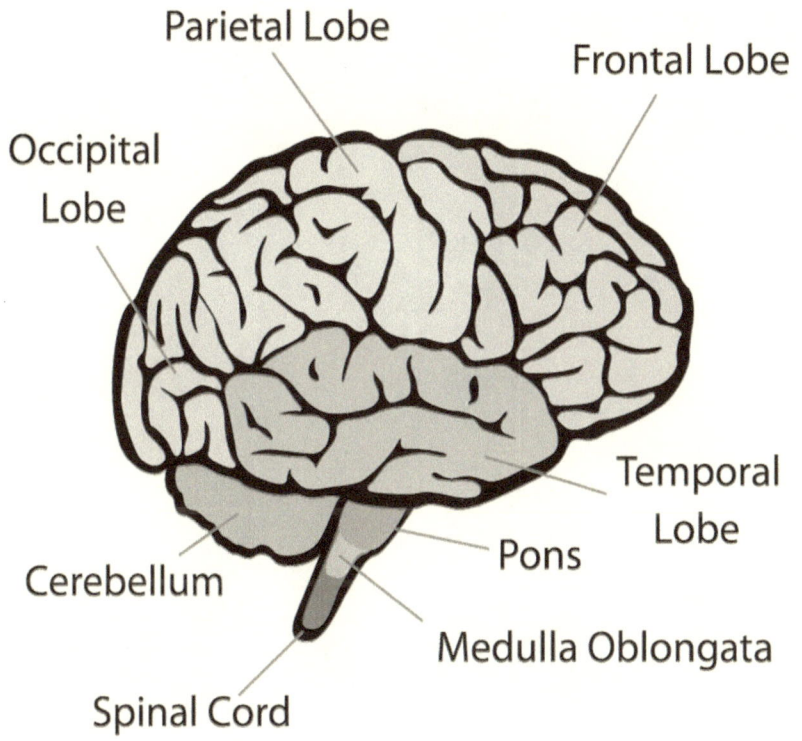

Parietal Lobe

Frontal Lobe

Occipital Lobe

Temporal Lobe

Cerebellum

Pons

Medulla Oblongata

Spinal Cord

BRAIN FUNCTION REVIEW

There are areas of the brain, called lobes, that generally are responsible for certain functions. Damage to any of these areas will cause functional and behavioral changes according to the primary functions of the affected lobe. This is a brief, general overview of these areas and what functions they contain:

1. Frontal lobe (located just behind your forehead)

    - Initiation
    - Mental reasoning and flexibility
    - Speaking
    - Organization/concentration
    - Problem-solving and self-monitoring behaviors
    - Judgment and safety awareness
    - Personality and emotional responses
    - Inhibition of behaviors
    - Planning and awareness of abilities and limitations

2. Temporal lobe (located just above and behind your ears on both sides)

    - Memory, both long term (what happened last month, ten years ago) and short term (what happened this morning or five minutes ago)
    - Understanding language, following verbal commands
    - Hearing
    - Organization and sequencing of tasks

3. Brain stem (at the base of the brain, back of the head as it goes into the neck)

   • Breathing
   • Sleeping/waking
   • Heart rate
   • Attention/concentration
   • Arousal/consciousness

4. Cerebellum (located at the back of the head)

   • Balance
   • Coordination both fine motor (hand/finger movements) and gross motor (arm and leg movements)
   • Skilled motor activity (handwriting, typing)

5. Occipital lobe (located in the back of the head)

   • Vision, both what you see and how you interpret what you see

6. Parietal lobe (located on the side of the head, above the temporal lobe toward the top of the head)

   • Sense of touch
   • Differentiation of items as to size, shape, color
   • Spatial perception (awareness of one's body in relationship to objects in the room)
   • Visual perception (identifying what you see, depth perception, and some visual memory)

PHYSICAL SIGNS YOU MAY SEE

Thinking

   • Short-term or long-term memory loss
   • Slow processing of what is heard with slow verbal response

- Difficulty concentrating or paying attention
- Unable to read or write
- Difficulty with depth perception or judging distance and impaired judgment
- Sensitivity to light
- Inability to follow either one-step or multistep commands

Physical signs

- Seizures
- Fatigue and need to take more frequent naps
- Sleep disturbances
- Visual impairments, double vision, blindness
- Loss of hearing or ringing in the ears
- Headaches
- Poor balance or decreased muscle/motor control
- Paralysis on one or both sides of the body

Emotional or behavioral signs

- Depression, grief, anxiety
- Low tolerance for stressful or noisy environments
- Inappropriate behaviors, like hitting, biting, kicking, or cursing
- Irritability, low frustration tolerance, anger
- Impulsivity or a lack of safety awareness or judgment
- Mood swings, such as laughing or crying excessively

Lateralization of Brain Functions

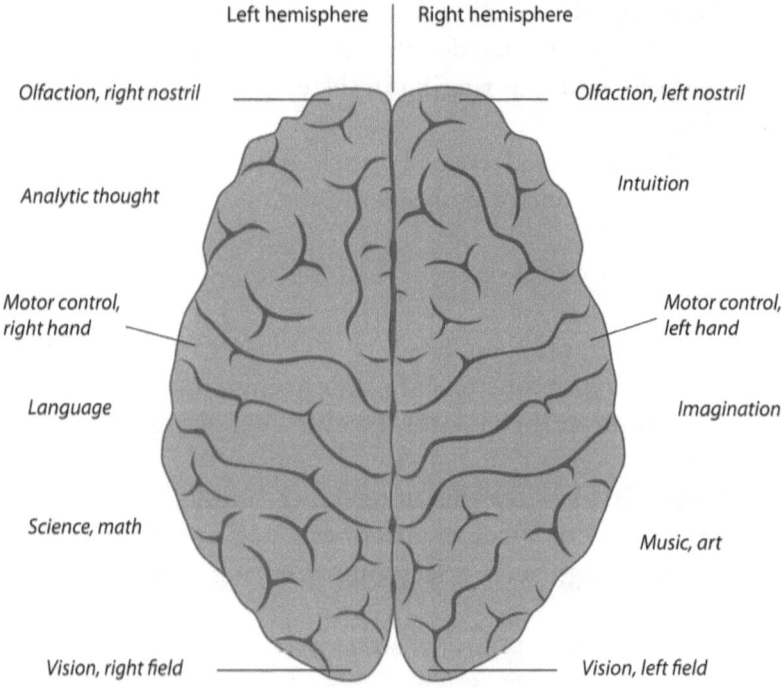

Left hemisphere | Right hemisphere

Olfaction, right nostril — — Olfaction, left nostril

Analytic thought

Intuition

Motor control, right hand

Motor control, left hand

Language

Imagination

Science, math

Music, art

Vision, right field — — Vision, left field

NOTES

THE INJURY

THE INJURY

So you received the word that your family member was injured and in the intensive care unit (ICU). Shock is the initial reaction that most families experience. As family and friends gather at the hospital, you are anxious to know what the status of your loved one is. Rest assured that medical personnel are doing all they can to stabilize your loved one, and their primary goal is the care of your family member. Also, be assured that as soon as they can come to give you a report on your loved one, they will contact you or find you in the waiting area. This may be a few hours to several hours. This can be a very stressful time for families. Common reactions are panic, anger, guilt, and feeling "numb." These are normal responses. Be sure to contact those family members or friends who can provide support for you during this waiting time. They can offer support and help the time to pass more quickly. It could be several hours before you are allowed to see your loved one. This is for their safety and continued emergency care. Hospital social workers and chaplains are available to assist you with your need for support. Please ask the admitting personnel to contact them for you.

THE INITIAL MEETING WITH THE DOCTOR

In a later section of this book, there are commonly used terms that your doctor may say to you during this initial visit and in the days to follow. If your doctor says a term you don't understand, please ask him/her to explain it to you. You may also write it down and look it up in the "terminology" section of this book. Realize that each person who has a brain injury responds differently and heals at different rates. Doctors and staff will be cautious with their prognosis and careful about giving families false hopes, so their initial information may be limited. This too can be frustrating for families. Recovery can take weeks or months, and it is impossible to say what the outcome will be at this early stage. Try to be patient, and realize that medical personnel cannot know if the individual will be able to return to a normal life at this early stage.

CODE WORD

You will need to establish a code word when calling in to check on your loved one. This is a requirement of the Health Insurance Portability and Accountability Act or HIPAA, so information about your loved one can only be shared with those who know the code word. It can be any word you choose, and you will need to let the nursing staff know what this is. Then only share this code word with those you want to have access to information about your loved one's status. Please share with others that if they call in to ask about your loved one and don't have the code word, medical personnel are not allowed by law to discuss anything about the patient. This is to preserve the patient's privacy and confidentiality.

ADVANCED DIRECTIVES

This allows a patient to make decisions regarding their own health care or name someone else to make health-care decisions if the patient becomes unable to make their own. This form can only be completed by patients who are alert and oriented. This includes consents for resuscitation should the need arise. Medical personnel will want to know if your family member has a "DNR/DNI" (do not resuscitate/do not intubate) order. If they do not or you don't know, the next of kin may be called upon to decide on this. Hospitals will have a form that they need you to fill out. It is a good idea to become familiar with a DNR or DNI consent. A helpful website for information is www.everydayhealth.com/brain-tumor/living-wills-and-advance-directives.aspx.

POWER OF ATTORNEY (POA)

This is a document needed for those patients who are unable to make medical decisions for themselves and are adults (over age eighteen in most states). This document can only be completed by individuals who are alert and oriented and able to make their own decisions. Families are encouraged to bring in any previously completed documents for POA upon admission to the hospital or as soon as possible. The social worker or the case manager for the ICU can provide you with information regarding the use and need for this document and required forms. (Forms can be downloaded for free at https://www.rocketlawyer.com.)

INSURANCE AND FUNDING ISSUES

The social worker for the ICU is the best person to contact early during your loved one's stay. This person can provide valuable information on insurance and funding and assist in applications for funding when needed. Ask nursing personnel to contact the social worker or the ICU case manager for you to assist you in the following:

- **Social Security Disability Insurance (SSDI)** is based upon an individual's work history. To qualify, it needs to be determined that the patient may be unable to work up to twelve months or more postinjury.
- **Social Security Income (SSI) supplement** is a federal program that is based upon income and assets and the patient's inability to work up to twelve months or more postinjury.
- **Institutional Medicaid** is a state program for individuals who meet income and residency qualifications and for patients needing an inpatient setting for thirty days or more.
- **Hospital care plans** are offered by some hospitals for low-income residents of the county where the hospital is located. Ask the unit case manager or the social worker if the hospital offers such a plan.

NOTES

ROLES OF MEDICAL PERSONNEL IN THE ICU

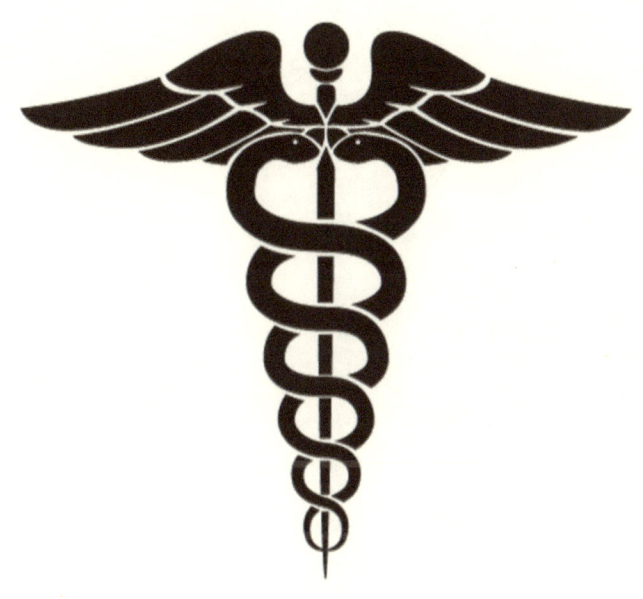

ROLES OF MEDICAL PERSONNEL IN THE ICU

(It may be helpful to keep a notebook with the names of people who work with your loved one for future reference.)

Occupational therapist (OT): Evaluates a patient's upper body function (hands, arms, fingers), eye–hand coordination, fine motor control, ability to do activities of daily living (ADLs; see above), and need for splints, exercises, evaluation of cognitive function, and adaptive equipment to help with independence (www.aota.org)

Physical therapist (PT): Evaluates muscle strength, muscle tone, endurance, general mobility in large muscle groups, range of motion, walking, transfers in/out of bed, and balance (www.apta.org)

Respiratory therapist (RT): Person responsible for the treatment or management of acute and chronic breathing disorders as through the use of respirators (ventilators) or the administration of breathing medications (www.aarc.org)

Nurses: Person responsible for administration of all medications, monitoring of body functions, and doing daily care. In the ICU, these will most likely be neuroscience nurses (aann.org).

Nurse techs: Assists the nurses with aspects of care including administering baths, emptying catheters, and changing bed linens.

Health unit clerk (HUC): Responsible for the paperwork involved in the daily operations of the ICU, including entering doctor's orders, assisting with chart/record management, directing phone calls.

Social worker (SW): Works with patients, other professionals, family member and funding sources to coordinate needed services, communicate with other medical personnel, assist in making discharge plans, and transitions from inpatient to outpatient community services. Some hospitals may call them case managers.

Laboratory technicians: Responsible for drawing blood and body fluid samples for testing as directed by physicians and nurses (www. americanmedtech.org)

Wound care nurses (WOC): Responsible for evaluating any skin wound and making recommendations as to the proper care and treatment of skin wounds (www.wocn.org)

Charge nurse: Per shift, responsible for the smooth organization of the unit, scheduling of nursing personnel, and interaction with physicians.

Unit director: Oversees the total unit, including all personnel, for administrative purposes

Intensivist: Doctor responsible for the medical status of the patient while in the ICU. This doctor will answer questions about medical issues that are not related to the brain condition. **Neurologist**: Doctor who specializes in treating diseases of the nervous system. His work may include seizure disorders, such as epilepsy; infections of the nervous system, including encephalitis, meningitis, or brain abscesses; neurodegenerative disorders, such as Lou Gehrig's disease, multiple sclerosis, and Alzheimer's disease; spinal cord disorders, including inflammatory and autoimmune disorders; and headaches, such as cluster headaches, migraines, and headaches of unknown origin. If your loved one had a stroke, this is the doctor you ask about issues with the stroke.

Neurosurgeon: Physician who specializes in the diagnosis and **surgical treatment** of disorders of the central and peripheral nervous system, including congenital anomalies, trauma, tumors, vascular disorders, infections of the brain or spine, stroke, or degenerative diseases of the spine. This is the doctor who operates on hemorrhages and aneurysms and performs other surgical procedures on the brain if needed.

NOTES

TERMINOLOGY

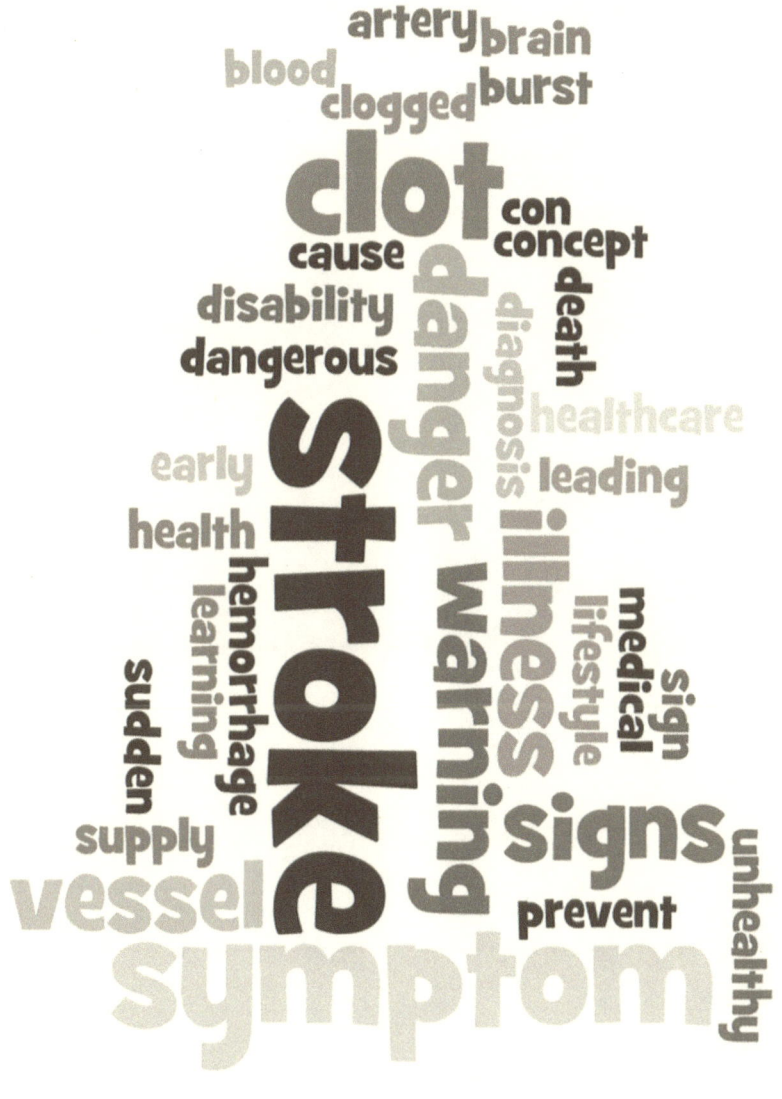

TERMINOLOGY

Acute care hospital: Inpatient medical care facility for short-term, acute medical needs.

Activities of daily living (ADLs): Routine daily activities including personal hygiene, such as bathing, dressing, feeding, and household management and job skills

Agnosia: When one fails to recognize familiar objects through the senses of taste, touch, vision, and hearing

Aneurysm (brain aneurysm, cerebral aneurysm): A bulging weakened formation on an artery, usually caused by hypertension, an excessive amount of fatty deposits, or weakness in the artery wall

Aneurysm clipping procedure: The procedure used to clip an aneurysm so it can be repaired or removed; also may use a coiling procedure that places a coil around the aneurysm to stabilize it

Anoxia: A lack of oxygen causing damage to parts of the brain

Aphasia: The loss of the ability to speak and/or to understand language

Apraxia: Difficulty doing complex or skilled movement involving hands as in fine motor movement or movements of the feet (for walking) or tongue (for speech and eating)

Aspiration: When fluid or food goes into the lungs, which can cause an infection or pneumonia; may be a result of poor coordination of the swallow response

Ataxia: Poor coordination of muscle movement, which may look like tremors (shakiness) with inability to manipulate objects or coordinate movements of the hands, feet, or trunk

Bronchoscopy: A procedure using a viewing tube to evaluate a patient's lung and airways, including the voice box and vocal cords, trachea, and many branches of the lungs.

CT scan: An imaging technique in which pictures of the brain are taken to detect tumors, hemorrhages, blood clots, abscesses, or abnormal findings. Dye may be injected into the patient's veins.

Carotid endarterectomy: A surgical procedure in which a doctor removes fatty deposits from one of the two main arteries in the neck supplying blood to the brain

Catheter (urinary): May also be referred to as a "Foley catheter"; a flexible tube inserted into the bladder for urine drainage

Cerebral vascular accident (CVA): Also known as a stroke, which is a sudden interruption in the blood supply of the brain (for types, see ischemic and hemorrhagic)

Chest tube: Chest drainage therapy is done to relieve pressure on the lungs and remove fluid that could promote infection. Installing a chest drainage tube can be either an emergency or a planned procedure.

Cognition: The conscious process of thinking, perception, memory, problem solving, understanding, and reasoning

Craniectomy: A surgical removal of a section of bone (bone flap) from the skull for the purpose of operating on the underlying tissues or relieving intracranial (within the skull) pressure, in which the bone flap is not replaced at the end of the procedure. Often, this flap of bone is stored in the abdomen of the patient to maintain blood flow and then can be replaced at a later time once intracranial pressures return to normal.

Cranioplasty: The surgical procedure where the bone flap that was removed and placed in the abdomen is now replaced on the skull. This may also be accomplished using artificial bone, mesh, or a steel plate.

Craniotomy: The surgical incision of the skull for the purpose of operating on the underlying tissues, which may be accompanied by insertion of a drainage tube

Decubitus (pressure sores): A pressure area, bedsore, or skin opening or breakdown because of pressure

Deep vein thrombosis (DVT): Blood clots that can form anywhere in the body but most commonly in the arms or legs

Do not resuscitate (DNR): Means do not resuscitate if patient stops breathing or heart stops beating

Do not intubate (DNI): Means that the patient does not want to be intubated with the breathing tube and hooked to an artificial ventilator device

Dysarthria: Difficulty in forming words, slurred speech, slow speech

Endotracheal tube (ET tube): A tube that serves as an airway and is inserted through the patient's mouth or nose, through the throat and vocal cords, and into the air passages to help breathing and is usually attached to a ventilator (portable breathing machine)

Family/caregivers: Mother/father, son/daughter, sister/brother, primary caregiver/significant other, aunt/uncle, cousins, or any other prespecified next of kin (NOK)

Family-centered care: The recognition that the family is the constant variable in a patient's life. For this reason, family-centered care is built on partnerships between families and professionals.

Fisher scale: A scale for grading CT scan appearance in patients with brain hemorrhages, with higher scores being more severe cases (Fisher & Kistler, 1980).

Description	Group
No subarachnoid blood detected	1
Diffuse subarachnoid blood or vertical layers of blood < 1 mm thick	2
Localized clots and/or vertical layers of blood < 1 mm thick	3
Intracerebral or intraventricular clots with diffuse or no subarachnoid blood	4

Flaccid: Lack of normal muscle tone; muscle appears flat and limp

Glasgow Coma Scale (GCS): Widely used scoring system to quantify level of consciousness following traumatic brain injury; scores range from 3 to 15, based on the sum of the best eye-opening response, the best verbal response, and the best motor response (The Internet Stroke Center, 2008)

Eye Opening (E)	Verbal Response (V)	Motor Response (M)
4=Spontaneous	5=Normal	6=Normal
3=To voice	4=Disoriented	5=Localizes to pain
2=To pain	3=Inappropriate	4=Withdraws to pain
1=None	2=Incomprehensible	3=Flexes to pain
	1=None	2=Extends to pain
		1=None
Total Score = **E+V+M**		

Pediatric Glasgow Coma Scale: Children (GCSC): Similar to the GCS described above but standardized for the pediatric population

Health Insurance Portability and Accountability Act of 2003 (HIPAA): Designed to protect medical records and other health information. The Department of Health and Human Services worked to create new standards that give patients increased control over how their records are used and who can access those records and more ability to protect individual privacy.

Hematoma: A collection of blood in tissues or spaces, which can be epidural (between the brain and its covering and under the skull), subdural (between the brain and its outer covering), or intracerebral (within the brain tissue)

Hemiparesis: Weakness on one side of the body

Hemiplegia: Paralysis on one side of the body

Hemorrhagic stroke: Also called intracerebral hemorrhage, occurs when a diseased or weakened blood vessel within the brain bursts, allowing blood to leak inside the brain.

Hunt and Hess scale: A scale for grading clinical status in patients with brain injuries that is widely used as a predictor of patient clinical outcomes (Hunt & Hess, 1968)

Description	Grade
Asymptomatic, mild headache, slight rigidity	1
Moderate to severe headache, rigidity, no neurologic deficit other than cranial nerve palsy	2
Drowsiness/confusion, mild focal neurologic deficit	3
Stupor, moderate–severe hemiparesis	4
Coma, decerebrate posturing	5

Hypoxic brain injury: Reduction in the supply of oxygen to the brain because of trauma or other causes such as respiratory arrest

Intracranial pressure (ICP): Pressure measured from a needle into the cerebral fluid, which monitors the pressure of the brain inside the skull. This is done with an extraventricular drain.

Inpatients: Persons admitted to the hospital with at least an overnight stay.

Intracerebral hemorrhage (ICH): Intracerebral hemorrhage occurs when a diseased or damaged blood vessel within the brain bursts, allowing blood to leak inside the brain. The sudden increase in pressure within the brain can cause damage to the brain cells surrounding the blood vessel. If the amount of blood increases rapidly, the sudden buildup of pressure can lead to unconsciousness or death.

Intraventricular hemorrhage (IVH): Bleeding in the ventricles of the brain, especially from fragile blood vessels in adults; may accompany intracerebral or subarachnoid hemorrhage

Intraparenchymal hemorrhage (IPH): Happens deep in the brain or cerebellum. These sites are all supplied by small penetrating arteries that are sensitive to the effects of increased blood pressure.

Ischemic stroke: Occurs when there is a blockage in an artery in the brain. If an artery is blocked, the cells called neurons cannot produce enough energy and will stop functioning. If this blockage lasts for more than a few minutes, the brain cells die.

Intravenous (IV): Tubing inserted into a vein for fluids and medications

Long-term acute care (LTAC): A placement recommendation when your family member may need more acute care for a longer period. Patients may need to breathe with a ventilator, have a tracheotomy that still requires regular suctioning, have wound care issues, and/or not be ready for rehabilitation.

Neurosciences intensive care unit (NSICU): Those patient units within the hospital designated as the highest level of direct medical care with staffing ratios of 1:2 (nursing personnel: patient). Patients in the NSICU are generally those who have suffered some kind of central nervous system event.

Nasogastric tube (NG tube): Inserted through the patient's nose and into the stomach for the purpose of giving nutrition for those patients who cannot or are unsafe to swallow food or fluids.

Occupational therapist (OT): Evaluates a patient's upper body function (hands, arms, fingers), eye-hand coordination, fine motor control, ability to do activities of daily living (ADLs; see above), and need for splints, exercises, evaluation of cognitive function, and adaptive equipment to help with independence (www.aota.org)

Percutaneous epigastric tube (PEG): Inserted directly into the stomach for the purpose of administering nutrition for those patients who cannot or are not safe to swallow foods or fluids for a longer period. These are reversible.

Physical therapist (PT): Evaluates muscle strength, muscle tone, endurance, and general mobility in large muscle groups, range of motion, walking, transfers in/out of bed, and balance (www.apta.org)

Ranchos Los Amigos Scale (RLA): Scored from I to VIII (www.rancho.org)

I. No response

- Does not respond to sound, sight, touch, or movement

II. Generalized response

- Begins to respond to sound, sight, touch, or movement
- Responds slowly, inconsistently, or after a delay
- Responds in the same way to what he hears, sees, or feels. Responses may include chewing, sweating, breathing faster, moaning, moving, and/or increasing blood pressure.

III. Localized response

- Awakes on and off during the day
- Makes more movements than before
- Reacts more specifically to what he sees, hears, or feels. For example, he may turn toward a sound, withdraw from pain, and attempt to watch a person move around the room.
- Reacts slowly and inconsistently
- Begins to recognize family and friends
- Follows some simple directions, such as "look at me" or "squeeze my hand"
- Begins to respond inconsistently to simple questions with "yes" or "no" head nods

IV. Confused, agitated

- Very confused and frightened
- Does not understand what he feels or what is happening around him
- Overreacts to what he sees, hears, or feels by hitting, screaming, using abusive language, or thrashing about. This is because of the confusion.
- Restrained, so he doesn't hurt himself
- Highly focused on his basic needs; i.e., eating, relieving pain, going back to bed, going to the bathroom, or going home
- May not understand that people are trying to help him
- Does not pay attention or be able to concentrate for a few seconds
- Has difficulty following directions
- Recognize family/friends some of the time
- With help is able to do simple routine activities, such as feeding himself, dressing, or talking

V. Confused, inappropriate, nonagitated

- Able to pay attention for only a few minutes
- Confused and has difficulty making sense of things outside himself
- Does not know the date, where he is, or why he is in the hospital

- Is not able to start or complete everyday activities, such as brushing his teeth, even when physically able. He may need step-by-step instructions.
- Becomes overloaded and restless when tired or when there are too many people around
- Has a very poor memory. He will remember past events from before the accident better than his daily routine or information he has been told since the injury.
- Tries to fill in gaps in memory by making things up (confabulation)
- May get stuck on an idea or activity (perseveration) and need help switching to the next part of the activity
- Focuses on basic needs, such as eating, relieving pain, going back to bed, going to the bathroom, or going home

VI. Confused, appropriate

- Somewhat confused because of memory and thinking problems. He will remember the main points from a conversation but forget and confuse the details. For example, he may remember he had visitors in the morning but forget what they talked about.
- Follows a schedule with some assistance but becomes confused by changes in the routine
- Knows the month and year, unless there is a serious memory problem
- Pays attention for about thirty minutes but has trouble concentrating when it is noisy or when the activity involves many steps. For example, at an intersection, he may be unable to step off the curb, watch for cars, watch the traffic light, walk, and talk at the same time.
- Brushes his teeth, gets dressed, feeds himself, etc. with help
- Knows when he needs to use the bathroom
- Does or says things too fast, without thinking first
- Knows that he is hospitalized because of an injury but will not understand all the problems he is having
- More aware of physical problems than thinking problems

- Associates his problems with being in the hospital and thinks he will be fine as soon as he goes home

VII.   Automatic, appropriate

- Follows a set schedule
- Able to do routine self-care without help, if physically able. For example, he can dress or feed himself independently, has problems in new situations, and may become frustrated or act without thinking first.
- Has problems planning, starting, and following through with activities
- Has trouble paying attention in distracting or stressful situations, for example, family gatherings, work, school, church, or sports events
- Does not realize how his thinking and memory problems may affect future plans and goals. Therefore, he may expect to return to his previous lifestyle or work.
- Continues to need supervision because of decreased safety awareness and judgment. He still does not fully understand the impact of his physical or thinking problems.
- Thinks slower in stressful situations
- Inflexible or rigid, and he may be stubborn. However, his behaviors are related to his brain injury.
- Able to talk about doing something but will have problems actually doing it

VIII.   Purposeful, appropriate

- Realizes that he has a problem in his thinking and memory
- Begins to compensate for his problems
- More flexible and less rigid in his thinking. For example, he may be able to come up with several solutions to a problem.
- Ready for driving or job training evaluation
- Able to learn new things at a slower rate
- Still becomes overloaded with difficult, stressful, or emergency situations

- Shows poor judgment in new situations and may require assistance
- Needs some guidance making decisions
- Has thinking problems that may not be noticeable to people who did not know the person before the injury

Rehabilitation (acute inpatient): Recommended by OTs, PTs, or SLPs for patients who are able to tolerate up to three to five hours of any combination of therapies spread throughout the day. These patients need very little, if any, nursing care. This is a transition period where patients stay at the facility prior to going home. Most centers will take patients who are at a RLA scale of IV or higher only (see Rancho Los Amigos Scale at www. rancho.org). Length of stay vary, may be from several days to several weeks.

Rehabilitation (outpatient): Patients ready to go home and have no nursing needs, can perform transfers with family members, and may need assistance to do activities of daily living (bathing, dressing) but also need to continue to work on rehabilitation goals by coming in to a center for treatment from home weekly.

Respiratory therapist (RT): Person responsible for the treatment or management of acute and chronic breathing disorders as through the use of respirators (ventilators) or the administration of breathing medications (www.aarc.org)

Sequential compression devices (SCDs): Wrapped around the patient's lower legs with alternating compression (squeezing) to prevent blood clots from forming while the patient is immobile (see DVT)

Skilled nursing facility (SNF) or intermediate level rehabilitation: Recommended by OTs, PTs, and SLPs when patients aren't quite ready for three to five hours of therapy per day but could tolerate a one to two hours of treatment per day. These patients need more nursing care than could be provided at home or in an acute rehabilitation center. These patients, under Medicare guidelines, may stay for up to twenty-one days and then be reevaluated for long-term care needs.

Social worker (SW): Works with patients, other professionals, family members, and funding sources to coordinate needed services, communicate with medical personnel, and assist in making discharge plans and transitions from inpatient hospital stay to other inpatient providers, as well as outpatient and community services (www. naswdc.org)

Spasticity (hypertonicity): Involuntary increase in muscle tension or tone where the muscle resists; movement seems "tight" or "rigid" like it is always contracting

Speech language pathologist (SLP): Evaluates language skills (both hearing/understanding and speaking), communication, swallowing, memory, problem solving, cognition, reading, and awareness of safety issues (www.asha.org)

Subarachnoid hemorrhage (SAH): Occurs when a blood vessel just outside the brain ruptures, and the area of the skull surrounding the brain (the subarachnoid space) rapidly fills with blood. High-resolution CT scanning correctly identifies more than 95 percent of SAH cases, with blood appearing in the subarachnoid spaces. CT angiogram or a cerebral angiogram is important to determine the origin of the SAH. "Thunderclap" headaches should be considered SAH until proven otherwise and evaluated by CT of the head with/without a spinal tap (lumbar puncture).

Subdural hematoma or subdural hemorrhage (SDH): A collection of blood in the subdural space following trauma or in elderly patients with cerebral atrophy or those with blood clotting abnormalities or hypertension

Tracheotomy (trache): A temporary surgical opening in the front of the throat that assists with breathing

Traumatic brain injury (TBI): A nondegenerative, noncongenital insult to the brain from an external mechanical force, possibly leading to permanent or temporary impairments of cognitive, physical, and psychosocial functions with an associated diminished or altered state of consciousness (www.biausa.org)

Ventriculostomy: A surgical procedure for measuring pressure within the brain by placing a device within one of the fluid filled spaces in the brain

Ventriculoperitoneal shunt (VP shunt): A surgical procedure to insert a catheter to relieve pressure on the brain by draining off the excess fluid to a cavity in the abdomen

Ventilator (respiratory "vent"): A piece of equipment responsible for assisting the patient with breathing. This piece of equipment is monitored closely by nursing personnel and the respiratory therapist (RT).

NOTES

FLOW SHEET OF POSSIBLE DISCHARGE OPTIONS AND NURSE-TO-PATIENT RATIOS

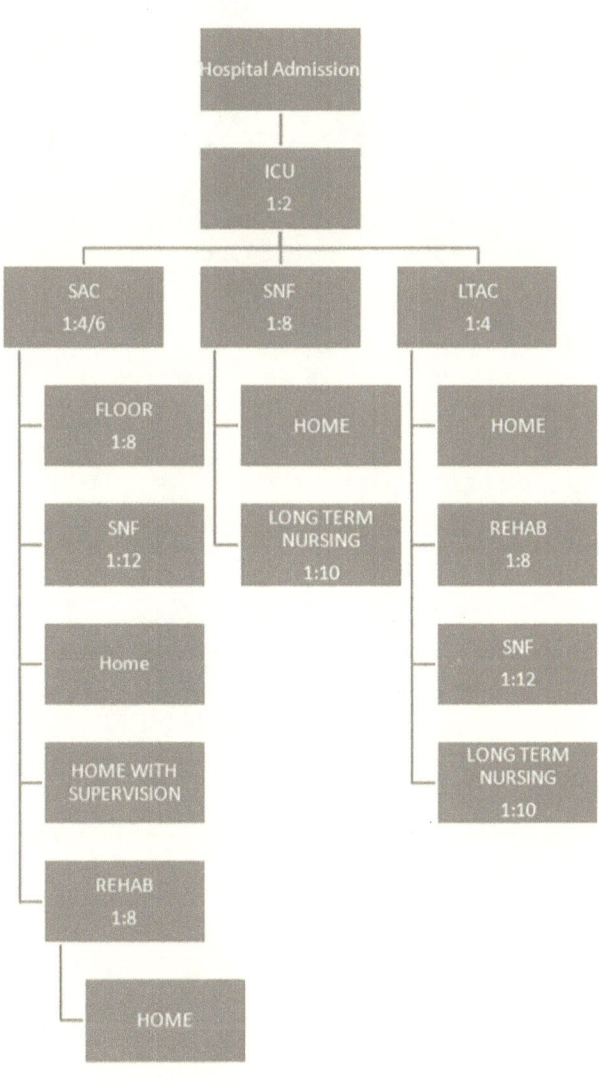

FREQUENTLY ASKED QUESTIONS FOR YOUR DOCTOR OR MEDICAL STAFF

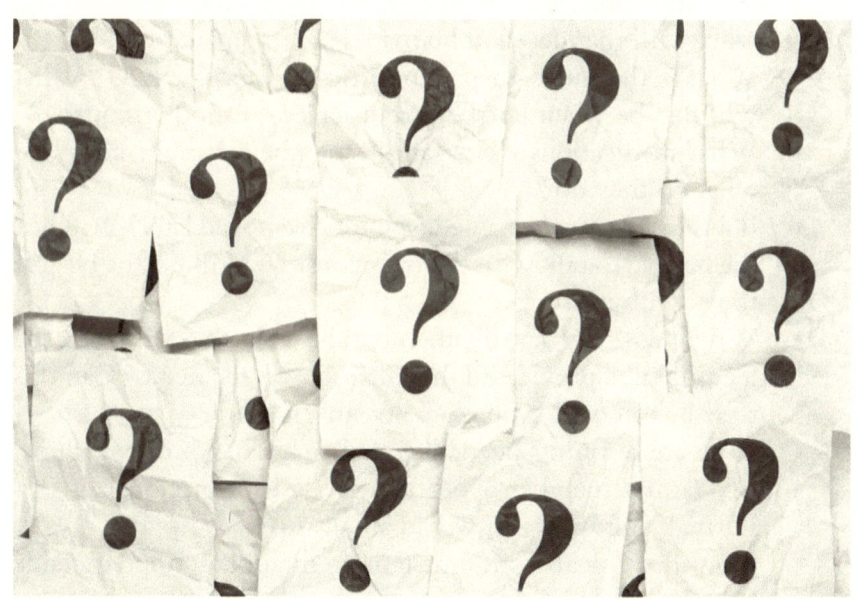

- What are your visitation policies and times?
- What time does the doctor come in each day so I can speak with him/her?
- What part of the brain has been damaged?
- What do these parts of the brain do?
- Who will help me with questions that I have?
- How will his/her memory or thinking be affected?
- What can I do to help him/her right now?
- Can someone help me with insurance or funding issues?
- Who will help with his/her rehabilitation?
- Will his/her rehabilitation be done here, and when will it start?
- Can someone from his/her family stay with him/her in the ICU?
- What are the visiting hours for the ICU?
- Will my family member be transferred to another floor, and when will that decision be made?
- What is the nurse-to-patient ratio here in the ICU? What will that be when he/she is transferred to another floor?
- What medications is my family member on right now, and what do they do?
- If a tracheotomy is needed, can it be removed later? Will he/she be able to talk with the tracheotomy? Will he/she be able to eat with it?
- When will my family member be able to eat? Does the feeding tube provide all the nutrition he/she needs? Can this tube be removed when he/she can eat again?
- Why are restraints needed to tie his/her hands down?
- My family member appears depressed (or anxious); is this normal, and what can we do about this?
- How do I deal with my family member's unpredictable behavior and agitation?
- What is the role of the physical therapist? Occupational therapist? Speech therapist? Social worker? Respiratory therapist?
- What is a long-term acute care (LTAC) placement, and can I have a list of places to visit?

- What is a skilled nursing facility (SNF), and can I have a list of places to visit?
- What rehabilitation centers are there in town, and can I have a list of places to visit?
- Who makes the arrangements (transportation, funding, etc.) for the transfer to another facility?
- How do I get copies of all the records from the hospital?
- Who do I talk to about applying for disability (SSI or SSDI) for my family member?
- Who do I talk to about lodging and meals for myself and my family while my family member is in ICU? Does the hospital have a discount agreement with any hotels nearby?
- Who do I talk to about family and medical leave (per FMLA) for my work/employer?
- Who do I talk to about applying for Medicare or Medicaid?
- Where do I find a bus schedule or map of the area and public transportation information?
- How can I get assistance with the cost of meals while I am here with my loved one?

NOTES

COMMUNITY AND
ONLINE RESOURCES

COMMUNITY RESOURCES

ELDERLY SERVICES

Department of Health and Human Services Office of Senior Affairs
www.hhs.gov

NATIONAL ORGANIZATIONS

Brain Injury Association of America
1608 Spring Hill Rd
Suite 110
Vienna VA 22182
braininjuryinfo@biausa.org
http://www.biausa.org
Tel.: 703-761-0750, 800-444-6443
Fax: 703-761-0755

Family Caregiver Alliance/National Center on Caregiving
785 Market St.
Suite 750
San Francisco CA 94103
info@caregiver.org
http://www.caregiver.org
Tel.: 415-434-3388, 800-445-8106
Fax: 415-434-3508

National Alliance for Caregiving
4720 Montgomery Lane, Second Floor
Bethesda MD 20814

info@caregiving.org
Tel.: 301-718-8444
Fax: 301-951-9067

National Association of State Head Injury Administrators
Tel.: 800-444-6443
www.nashia.org

National Rehabilitation Information Center (NARIC)
8201 Corporate Drive
Suite 600
Landover MD 20785
naricinfo@heitechservices.com
http://www.naric.com
Tel.: 301-459-5900, 301-459-5984 (TTY), 800-346-2742
Fax: 301-562-2401

National Stroke Association
9707 E Easter Lane
www.stroke.org
Englewood CO 80112
Tel.: 303-649-9299, 800-787-6537

National Spinal Cord Injury Association
6701 Democracy Blvd. Suite 300-9
Bethesda MD 20817
www.spinaldord.org

National Center on Shaken Baby Syndrome
2955 Harrison Blvd Suite 102
Ogden UT 84403
www.dontshake.com
Tel.: 801-627-3399, 888-273-0071

HELPFUL WEBSITES

Traumatic Brain Injury: Resources for Veterans with TBI
www.maketheconnection.net/TBI

Medical Equipment Information
http://www.medicare.gov/what-medicare-covers/part-b/durable-medical-equipment.html

Head Trauma Resource
www.braininjury.com

The Brain Trauma Foundation
https://www.braintrauma.org/

Brain Injury Association of America
www.biausa.org/

National Institute of Neurological Disorders and Stroke
http://www.ninds.nih.gov/disorders/tbi/org_tbi.htm

NOTES

REFERENCES

Answers.com. (2008). *Respiratory Therapy*. Retrieved October 14, 2008, from Answers Corporation website: http://www.answers.com/topic/respiratory-therapy

Biology Online. (3). *VP Shunt*. Retrieved October 14, 2008, from Scientific American Partner Network website: http://www.biology-online.org/dictionary/Vp_shunt

Fisher C., Kistler J., Davis J. (1980). "Relation of cerebral vasospasm to subarachnoid hemorrhage visualized by computerized tomographic scanning." *Neurosurgery* 6 (1): 1–9.

Pietro, M. A. (2013). Neurologist. Retrieved from http://www.healthline.com/health/neurologist#TreatmentAreas2

Hunt W. E., Hess R. M. "Surgical risk as related to time of intervention in the repair of intracranial aneurysms." *Journal of Neurosurgery* 1968 Jan; 28(1):14–20.

Johnson, G. (2002–2008). *While you were waiting . . . The Rancho Los Amigos Scale*. Retrieved October 14, 2008, from The Waiting.com website: http://www.waiting.com/rancholosamigos.html

New Mexico Brain Injury Association. (2008). *New Mexico brain injury resource manual* (Spring 2008 ed.) [Brochure]. Santa Fe, NM: NM Aging and Long Term Services Department and the NM Brain Injury Advisory Council.

Rancho Los Amigos National Rehabilitation Center (2009). *Family guide to the rancho levels of cognitive functioning*. Retrieved from: http://rancho.org

Shifman and Stoppler. (2008). *Bronchoscopy*. Retrieved October 14, 2008, from MedicineNet.com website: http://www.medicinenet.com/bronchoscopy/article.htm#1whatis

Washington University. (1997–2008). *The Internet Stroke Center.* Retrieved October 14, 2008, from Washington University website: http://www.strokecenter.org/

Webmd. (2005). *Traumatic brain injury.* Retrieved October 14, 2008, from WebMD, LLC website: http://www.webmd.com/

www.ingramcontent.com/pod-product-compliance
Lightning Source LLC
Chambersburg PA
CBHW021024180526
45163CB00005B/2107